Energy

Ultimate Energy
Discover How To Increase Your Energy Levels Using The Best All Natural Foods, Supplements And Strategies For A Life Full Of Abundant Energy

By Ace McCloud
Copyright © 2014

Disclaimer

The information provided in this book is designed to provide helpful information on the subjects discussed. This book is not meant to be used, nor should it be used, to diagnose or treat any medical condition. For diagnosis or treatment of any medical problem, consult your own physician. The publisher and author are not responsible for any specific health or allergy needs that may require medical supervision and are not liable for any damages or negative consequences from any treatment, action, application or preparation, to any person reading or following the information in this book. Any references included are provided for informational purposes only. Readers should be aware that any websites or links listed in this book may change.

Table of Contents

Introduction 6
Chapter 1: Why is Energy So Important? 7
Chapter 2: Best Proven Natural Methods for Boosting Your Energy 8
Chapter 3: Eat, Drink, and Be Energized 14
Chapter 4: All Natural Vitamins and Supplements for Energy 25
Chapter 5: Living One Super-Energizing Life 30
Conclusion 32
My Other Books and Audio Books 33

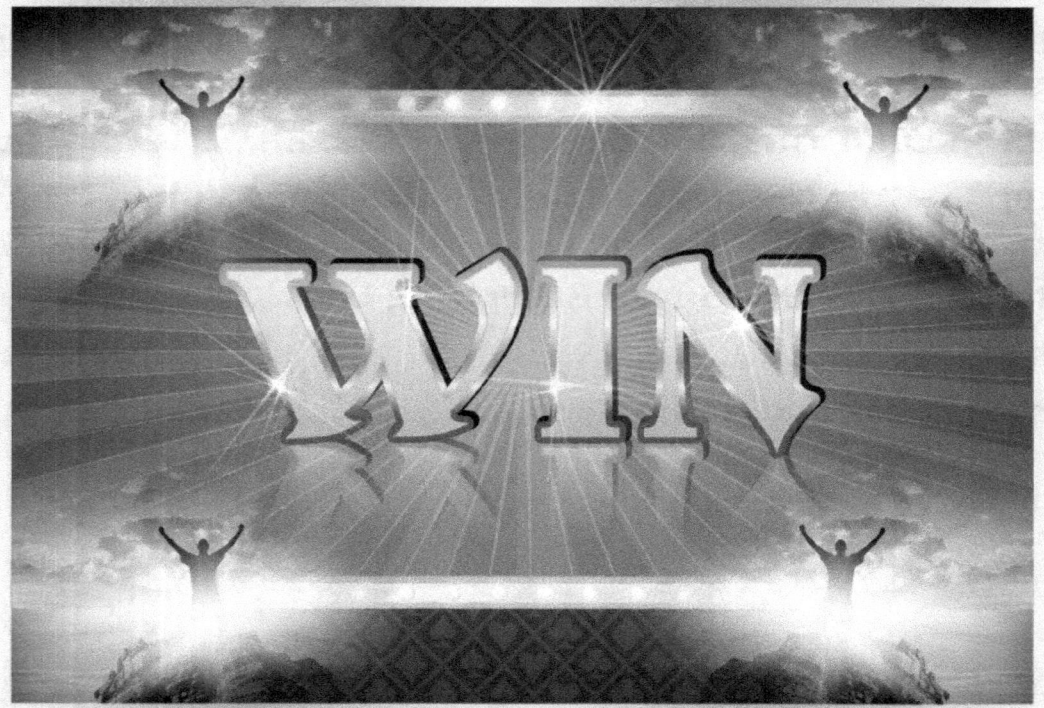

Be sure to check out my website for all my Books and Audio books.

www.AcesEbooks.com

Introduction

I want to thank you and congratulate you for buying the book, "Ultimate Energy: Strategies To Increase Your Energy Levels, All Natural Methods For Gaining Energy, The Best Foods and Supplements For Improved Energy, And Living An Energy Boosting Lifestyle ."

This book has everything you need to dramatically raise your natural energy levels. Do you often feel tired and sluggish a couple of hours after first waking up? Do you lie down on the couch after work with the intentions of taking a nap and then end up sleeping for hours? Do you wish that you had more energy to spend more time with your friends and family? If you have answered "yes" to one or more of these questions, your problems are finally over. This book will help you discover the **right** ways to boost the levels of energy in *your* body. Whether it's some simple changes in your daily routine, watching what you eat, or learning what kind of nutrients that your body needs for more energy, this book will guide you down the right path. Life is far too precious to be spending it tired and exhausted all the time! You will be shocked at what a few simple changes in your diet and lifestyle can do for the quality and energy levels of your life. If you're ready to live a life full of abundant energy, then keep on reading!

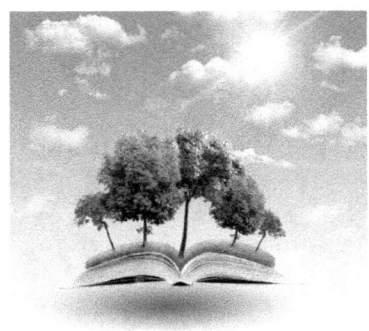

Chapter 1: Why is Energy So Important?

Energy is something that we use constantly—after all, it's what drives and motivates us! You may not know it, but you use energy every day, whether you are studying, thinking, moving something, playing a sport, or even growing. Without energy, we tend to feel tired, sluggish, unproductive, and unmotivated. Low levels of energy make us want to lie in bed all day and do nothing. Energy helps us keep our minds clear, focused, and on track with our goals. Without it, our lives do not have a clear direction. Therefore, having a healthy level of energy is essential for living a happy, productive, and fulfilling life. Our energy levels depend on the food we eat and the way we take care of our bodies. People with high levels of energy often function better than people with low levels of energy.

Having low levels of energy can cause us to live an unhealthy lifestyle. First and foremost, low levels of energy cause fatigue. When we suffer from fatigue, our work doesn't get done, whether at home, school, or work. Fatigue also causes us to make unhealthy eating decisions because we won't feel motivated to prepare a healthy meal with fresh ingredients—we will most likely order out from a fast food restaurant or cook something out of a can, which is usually loaded with sodium and other unhealthy additives. An unhealthy diet can also limit our intake of iron, vitamin B12, magnesium, and fatty acids, all of which provide our bodies with healthy nutrients that it transforms into energy.

Low levels of energy also make us more tired and more tempted to drink energy drinks or sodas, both of which are artificial products that are loaded with sugar and caffeine, which can give a quick boost of energy, but actually cause our energy levels to crash later on, the opposite effect of what we want. It is easily possible to become addicted to caffeine and sugar, which can lead to even more health problems. Not having enough energy in your body also leads to a decreased work ethic, a lost interest in hobbies, and less time with your family or friends.

This book looks to be the answer in helping you increase your energy in sustainable ways that leave you healthier and happier in the long run. You will learn some natural methods for boosting your energy that you can work into your daily routine. In the coming chapters you will also learn about the top foods that you can eat for energy, as well as how to turn them into ultimate, energizing recipes. This book also contains a list of the top 15 best, all-natural vitamins and supplements that you can take to bring a little more energy into your life, especially if you have any nutrient deficiencies. Finally, you will learn how to combine all these measures to efficiently live a fully-charged life, which will benefit you for years to come.

Chapter 2: Best Proven Natural Methods for Boosting Your Energy

When you're constantly on the go, as many people are today, it is sometimes hard to keep yourself energized. Artificial energy drinks and candy bars easily tempt us as quick, cheap, and easy ways to stay energized. I used to use them all the time as my main source of energy, when I was on the go. However, they did not seem to have a positive effect on me. While I enjoyed the initial surge of energy, I often found myself crashing and even more tired and dehydrated later on. Sometimes it would take me a full day or two to recover from just one day of sodas, energy drinks, and other quick energy sources. While I was able to get a lot done in the initial burst of energy, I could have been much more productive and healthy over the long term if I had just done things right. I have discovered that the best ways to keep your body full of energy is to use all-natural products and remedies.

We all lead busy lives. No matter what kind of life you have, you probably have many responsibilities. If you're a businessperson, chances are that you are constantly thinking about your business, your clients, and the work that you have to do. If you're a parent, you probably use most of your time cleaning, cooking, and looking after your kids. Everyone's lives are different but one thing that we all have in common is a limited amount of time. Our many responsibilities often cause us to put a good night's sleep on the back burner. This is the first mistake that many people tend to make. Sleep is critical to having a healthy and energized life.

Sleep allows your brain and cells and other body cells to rest and charge back up for the next day. Your body also releases healthy hormones while your brain and cells rest. Although many of us believe that eight hours is the standard for sleeping, the amount of time needed for a good night's sleep actually depends on our age. While babies need the most amount of time for sleep (16 hours), toddlers and adolescents aged 3 to 12 usually only need 10 or so hours of sleep. Many doctors recommend 8 hours of sleep for those aged 19 to 55 and people over 65 usually only need 6 hours of sleep. Surprisingly, 71% of people have reported that they do not get a standard amount of sleep and are actually sleep deprived.

If you consider yourself one of those people who do not get a good night's sleep, there are several steps that you can take to change that. The first step that you can take to ensure a good night's sleep is to make sure that you have the proper kind of bedding. Make sure that your pillow is firm and supports your head. Some pillows can aggravate your allergies because of the filling or dust mites that build up on the surface, which can disrupt the amount of sleep you may get. If you are allergic to the stuffing in your pillow, a non-allergenic pillow might be a good option for you. I highly recommend the **Sleep Innovations Reversible 2-in-1 Bed Pillow**. Instead of traditional stuffing, this pillow contains hypoallergenic memory foam, which provides maximum comfort and does not affect allergies. If you are happy with the pillow that you have, I recommend getting a pillow case. Another great product is the **Allersoft 100-Percent Cotton Dust Mite & Allergy Control Pillow Encasement**. This pillow case is made from 100% cotton and will protect you from dust mites or anything else that may cause you to have an allergic reaction or otherwise disrupt your sleeping habits.

A second step that you can take to get a good night's sleep is to expose yourself to more light during the day. Make it a habit to open your shades as soon as you wake up to let the sun shine through. Try not to wear sunglasses during the day and spend whatever time you can outside. For example, you can gain more exposure to more light by eating your lunch outside or taking a short morning walk. If you absolutely cannot spend much time outside (or if it's too cold out) you can keep your blinds and shades open to let more sunlight into your house or, if you spend a lot of time at work, you could try to move your desk closer to a window. If, for some reason, you are unable to spend a lot of time outside, you can use a light therapy box as a way to get a good amount of light exposure. One great light box product is the **NatureBright SunTouch Plus Light and Ion Therapy Lamp**. This lamp is safe, effective, and will have you feeling like you've been lying in the sun all day, even if the skies are overcast.

Although more exposure to light during the day is good for getting enough sleep, you should also take steps to get less exposure to light at night, especially when you're getting ready for bed. At night, your body produces melatonin, a natural hormone that helps you fall asleep. Too much light exposure affects how much melatonin your body produces. You can help your body produce more melatonin by turning off all electronics at night, including your computers and televisions, reading from physical books instead of e-readers (the back light will affect your body's production of melatonin), and by turning off all your lights. If you are the type of person who likes to fall asleep with the television on in the background, try substituting it for soft music or a "book on tape."

It is also a great idea to have a comfortable bed. I have had a **Select Comfort Air Bed** for over seven years and it is awesome. I sleep great and wake up with no neck or back pain. I have tried all sorts of mattresses and I think the air beds are by far the best.

A good night's sleep is a key step for feeling more energized. More energy gained from sleeping will make you more productive, sharp, and emotionally settled during the day. If you are unable to get a good night's sleep, (for example, if you're woken up in the middle of the night due to an emergency) one way to make up for lost sleep is to take a mid-day nap. Not only is sleep great for re-energizing yourself, but it also protects you from other health issues because it boosts your immune system. Some newer studies have shown that sleep deprivation can now lead to heart disease, diabetes, and other diseases.

Another great, all-natural way to boost your levels of energy is to exercise. Exercise promotes high levels of energy because it stimulates our natural hormones, strengthens our hearts over time (the more blood our hearts pump through our body, the more energy we will have), and good exercise habits can even lead to getting a good night's sleep. Research has shown that adults who exercise for at least 20 minutes a day for at least three times a week felt higher levels of energy and rarely felt tired or sluggish throughout the day. Exercise is also great for ensuring strong muscles and an overall feeling of wellness.

Almost any type of exercise will help you to become and stay energized. There are many energy-boosting exercises that are simple to do, even for those who do not regularly exercise or do not have a lot of time to exercise.

The easiest type of energy-boosting exercise is to take a brisk walk. It doesn't require much more than a pair of good walking shoes and a place to walk. If you consistently take brisk walks, your levels of energy will gradually overpower your levels of fatigue. Walking will also boost your levels of self-esteem, which will make you more motivated and energized. Walking outside also exposes you to sunlight, which can help you get a better night's sleep, so it's almost like a 2-in-1 routine. It is important to note that there is a certain technique to brisk walking. This YouTube video by Shawn Shawket **The Correct Way to Brisk Walking for Better Health** explains some of the proper techniques for brisk walking.

Walking is my favorite form of exercise. It is easy to do, you almost never get injured doing it, you get great results from it, and you can practice saying positive affirmations in your head while doing it along with various breathing techniques. A good breathing technique I learned from Tony Robbins was to quickly breath in four times through your nose in one complete inhalation, and then to breath out through your mouth four times quickly in one big exhalation. You can do this five to ten times to really get a boost of oxygen into your body. An example of a positive affirmation you can say while walking or almost anytime is: "I am super strong, happy, healthy, wealthy, and wise." Feel free to make up your own affirmations tailored to your specific strengths, desires and goals.

Deep breathing is another great exercise technique for boosting energy. Taking breaths that are too shallow prevent oxygen from flowing into the body and can lead to tension and stress. Deep breaths will help your heart pump more oxygen to your brain. Like brisk walking, there is a certain technique to deep breathing. One good way to practice deep breathing is to slowly inhale, hold it for four seconds and then exhale even more slowly. You can repeat this exercise a few times until you begin to feel relaxed and energized. This YouTube video, **How to Do Breathing Exercises: Meditation with Deep Breathing** by expertvillage, is a great example on how to practice deep breathing.

Stretching exercises are also a great way to increase your levels of energy. One stretch, known as the Virasana yoga pose, is great supplementary exercise to deep breathing. For this stretch, you should kneel on the floor, keeping your buttocks near your feet and your spine parallel to the floor. While joining your hands together in front of you, point your palms away from your face and raise them. Hold that position for one minute and breathe steadily. Do not hold the position for more than five minutes. When you're done, slowly bring your arms down and stand up, using your hands for support.

Some people may prefer to engage in aerobic exercise as a way to stay energized. Some good ways to use aerobics for boosting energy levels are to jump rope or to do push-ups or crunches. Finally, one "fun" way to get in some aerobic exercise is to turn up some music and dance. Creative dancing will increase your heart rate and give you many of the other benefits of intense aerobic exercises. It's also a great stress reliever, which can make you feel good about yourself and boost your energy levels even higher.

In addition to getting enough rest and exercise, there are some relaxation techniques that you can use to boost your levels of energy. Relaxation reduces stress, which can easily drain your energy. By being able to relax, you can increase your levels of energy and even be able to focus more clearly. You can't totally avoid stress, and some stress is even healthy, but there are some natural relaxation techniques that you can use to help keep your stress levels down and your energy levels up. An incredible way to reduce stress and increase the amount of joy in your life is through laughter therapy. If you would like to know more about this, be sure to check out my bestselling book: **Laughter and Humor Therapy**.

One of the most popular mental relaxation techniques is aromatherapy. Aromatherapy is the use of scented oils that help us relax by stimulating the part of the brain that controls our sense of smell. Many people use different aromatherapy techniques, depending on their preferences and situation. Some people directly inhale the oil, others let it evaporate into the air around them, and some even put the oil on their skin. Many people use aromatherapy to reduce anxiety, stress, sleep deprivation, and depression, all of which can lead to low levels of energy. Different combinations of oil create different scents and stimulate different moods. Some of my favorite essential oils I will put near my work station and just inhale them directly. This allows them to last an extremely long time and you get a good quick dose of aroma therapy. However, it is also nice when you can fill up a whole room with incredible scents for hours at a time.

Some of the best energy-boosting aroma therapy oils for stimulating your mind are **Lemon**, **Orange**, **Peppermint**, **Aniseed**, **Clove**, **Rosemary**, **Sandalwood**, and **Patchouli**. Aroma therapy oils that are best for stimulating the body are **Petitgrain**, **Peppermint**, **Tea Tree**, **Black Pepper**, **Juniper**, **Rosemary**, **Rose**, **Patchouli**, and **Ginger**. **Bergamot**, **Thyme**, **Pine**, **Rose**, **Rosewood**, and **Sandalwood** are also good oils for stimulating emotions.

The most popular way to use aromatherapy oils is to burn them in a candle or heat diffuser but there are several other ways to use them. You can add the oil to a spray bottle filled with water and use that as an air freshener. You can also add the oil to the hot wax of a candle, or combine them with your favorite lotion.

My personal favorite way of enjoying aromatherapy is with this [Armoma Therapy Essential Oil Diffuser](). It is a bit expensive, but after trying the various heat methods of diffusing the essential oils and being very disappointed, I got this model and it works great by steadily putting a mist of water and essential oils into the air. The auto shutoff feature and the fact that it glows several different colors is nice as well. The only drawback is that you can't use citrus oils in it such as lemon and orange because they tend to damage the unit.

Aromatherapy is a great way to relax, reduce mental stress, and boost your levels of energy. This short YouTube video posted by Howcast gives a great overview of how to use aromatherapy and how it can increase energy levels, [How to Use Aromatherapy's Essential Oils to Improve Your Life]().

Another all-natural, mental energy-boosting technique is meditation. Meditation involves learning how to focus your attention on something by keeping an open mind and a relaxed posture. Meditation helps stimulate relaxation and good health. Many people practice meditation as a way to reduce their levels of stress, anxiety, depression, and insomnia, all of which can drain one's energy.

A typical meditating session takes about 20 minutes out of your day. First, you should have a special room or place to meditate. The location you choose to meditate in should be quiet, peaceful, and private. Next, sit in a comfortable position with a straight back. You can sit in any position you like, as long as your back is straight. Set a timer for 20 minutes so you will not be preoccupied with keeping track of your time. Next, close your eyes and start focusing on your breaths. Then, start focusing your thoughts on relaxation. If you begin thinking of anything else, slowly bring yourself back to concentrating on relaxing. Meditation will help you balance your emotions and clear your mind. This YouTube video, [How to meditate](), by Rohit.Sharma is a great beginner's guide on meditation.

Another mentally relaxing, energy-boosting technique that you can try is massage therapy. Massages have been a method of healing for centuries. Many people find the sensation of touch calming and soothing. Now, there is scientific evidence that massages are a great healing method. A massage can lower your levels of anxiety and induce relaxation. It also increases blood circulation, cuts your levels of fatigue, and helps you sleep better, all of which contribute to higher levels of energy. An increased blood circulation helps more oxygen flow into your body and releases natural hormones that stimulate pleasure. A massage can take away any stress that can deprive you of a good night's sleep or energy in general. It can also aid in the healing of injuries and even help prevent injuries from happening. If you can't afford to pay for massages or don't have a loved one who can do this for you, you can always self-massage. For a great book on massage therapy, check out my book: **The Best Of Massage Therapy, Trigger Point Therapy, And Acupressure**.

These all-natural approaches to boosting your energy are great because they don't require drugs or medicine, they are free (unless you go to the gym to exercise or decide to buy oils for aromatherapy), and they are simple. Start out by focusing on getting a good night's sleep—the rest of the techniques work great as well, but they all come back to getting a good night's sleep. By combining all or some of these methods, you will be feeling full of energy in no time.

Chapter 3: Eat, Drink, and Be Energized

One of the best ways to naturally boost your energy is to eat foods that your body will turn into long-lasting bursts of energy throughout the day. Without any food at all, our bodies will get weak and become unable to function sharply. Once you have eaten something healthy and if you haven't eaten too much, then it's not long before you will feel stronger, able to think more clearly, and have the ability to work harder. However, what you eat depends on what kind of energy you will get. If you are like many people, the first type of energy food source you are probably thinking of is an energy drink or bar because they are fast, cheap, easy, and marketed to us in a sense that can make people believe that they are good for you. Contrary to popular belief, those food sources can actually leave you even more tired hours after consumption and can even have adverse effects on your heart. If you are at all worried about your heart health, you can check out my book: **Heart Disease Cure**. The rest of this chapter will outlines the top 30 energy "super-foods" that you can eat for breakfast, lunch, dinner, or as a snack to ensure a healthy, natural energy boost.

Tips for Eating

- Always make breakfast a priority every day, because it is the first way your body will refill with nutrients. My breakfast consists of a fruit and vegetable smoothie 95% of the time. I will drink a large glass of water first thing in the morning, have the smoothie after a quick stretching routing, and then drink another glass of water along with some of my favorite supplements like **Focus Formula**, **Licorice Root**, **Bee Caps**, **Vitamin B-12**, **Oatstraw**, and a variety of other great energy supplements we will discuss later in the book.
- Instead of eating 3 standard meals a day, try to eat 4 to 5 meals over the day. This will help keep you full and energetic from morning to night without being weighed down by excess food consumption. I wish I would have incorporated this strategy earlier in my life, as it makes a huge positive difference. Smaller, healthier meals is by far the best way to go and is done by the majority of pro athletes and peak performance specialists all over the world.
- Stay away from processed foods and refined sugars.
- Eat your meals within 5 hours of each other.
- Drink plenty of water to keep your body refreshed and hydrated. After many years and spending hundreds of dollars on a variety of different water products, I have finally concluded that the **ZeroWater** system is one of the best. It does an incredible job of filtering the water and leaving nothing behind but pure, great tasting water.
- Stay away from energy drinks, sodas, sugary sports drinks, or vitamin waters.

- Some of the best nutrients for your body are proteins, <u>B vitamins</u>, **Fiber**, <u>Iron</u>, <u>Magnesium</u>, <u>Vitamin A</u>, <u>Vitamin C</u>, <u>Vitamin E</u>, <u>Manganese</u>, and <u>Omega Fatty Acids</u>.

Breakfast

Breakfast is the most important meal of the day, although many people tend to think of it as the least important meal of the day. Eating a great breakfast that is healthy gives your body all the energy that it needs to get you through the day. It also keeps you full until snack or lunch time. Breakfast also helps you start your day off on a positive vibe, which will help you stay motivated and utilize positive energy throughout your day. Besides the smoothies I mentioned earlier, what kinds of breakfast foods are best for increasing your energy?

Eggs

Eggs are a common breakfast item and a great source of protein. Protein keeps your heart and immune system strong and healthy, which in turn gives your body more energy to use during the day. Eggs also provide your body with a great amount of energy because they do not interfere with your levels of blood sugar. They also contain Vitamins B12 and B6, which are great sources of natural energy because they help your body convert molecules into energy and help power your brain. Eggs are a popular source of early-morning energy because you can prepare them in many different ways. You can scramble them, cook them "sunny side up," boil them, or add them in an omelet.

Whole Grain Oatmeal

Whole grain oatmeal is another popular breakfast food that provides us with a good source of natural energy. Whole grains contain healthy carbohydrates, which help regulate our body cells for better levels of energy. Whole grains are also easier for our bodies to digest. Our bodies digest whole grains slower than grains that contain processed carbohydrates, so our bodies get an extra dose of energy from the difference in digestion. Oatmeal is an easy meal to prepare in the microwave or on the stovetop. For an extra healthy, energetic breakfast, top your oatmeal off with fruits or nuts, both of which also serve as great sources of energy.

Bran Cereal

Bran cereal is a great source of early-morning energy and it's also easy to prepare. Bran cereals are well-known for their high levels of fiber, which our bodies can digest easily, but they also contain high levels of protein, iron, magnesium, B Vitamins, and Vitamins A and C. Iron is a mineral in our bodies that helps our inner-body parts, like our lungs, to function. The better we can breathe, the more energy we will have. Magnesium is another mineral that helps our bodies utilize proteins and energy. To eat bran cereal, simply pour some in a bowl over skim milk or eat it dry. You can even add bananas to it for an extra serving of delicious fiber.

Quinoa

Many people call quinoa a "super food" because it is plant-based and contains high levels of all the amino acids that your body needs to get from a secondary food source. As a result, it is a food that is great for increasing your levels of energy because amino acids support proteins and can help stop our bodies from becoming drained of energy. For breakfast, you can make porridge out of plain quinoa by mixing it with water or skim milk. You can also add fresh fruit to the quinoa porridge or you can add the porridge to some plain yogurt.

Whole Grain Bread

Whole grain bread is a healthy, energizing alternative to white bread. Although both types of bread have similar calorie counts, whole grain bread has "better" calories than white bread. Whole grain bread also contains bran, which gives it a high content of fiber. Whole grain bread also contains more proteins, good carbohydrates, and vitamins than white bread. You can toast a slice or two of whole grain bread for a quick breakfast. You can make it even more energizing by adding some natural peanut butter or fresh fruit on the side. Wash it down with a glass of water or skim milk for a healthy, energizing breakfast.

Lunch and Dinner

Cardamom

Cardamom is an Asian spice that people often use for making curry, chai tea, or several other Asian cuisine dishes. Cardamom encourages blood flow and circulation by expanding your blood vessels. Better blood flow and circulation leads to increased amounts of energy. You can add cardamom to almost any dish for a spicy seasoning.

Brown Rice

Brown rice is a great side dish for many lunch and dinner meals and is also a great source of energy. Brown rice contains high levels of a nutrient called manganese. Manganese works with the proteins and carbohydrates in our bodies to create extra energy. You can eat brown rice by itself for a quick snack or you can have it as a side dish with salmon, lean pork, lean meat, or with fresh vegetables for a healthy, energizing meal.

Sweet Potatoes

Not only are sweet potatoes a great source of energy but they are a great way to get your kids to eat healthy too. Aside from their sweet taste, sweet potatoes contain high levels of Vitamins A and C, two vitamins that our bodies can use to make energy. You can use sweet potatoes for mashed potatoes, french fries, or just as a general side vegetable.

Lean Pork or Beef

Lean meats like pork or beef are a great way for meat lover's to make their levels of energy higher. Like quinoa, lean pork contains all the amino acids that our bodies need from secondary sources. 100 grams of lean pork also contains 30 grams of protein, 70% of Vitamin B12, 15% of iron, 10% of magnesium, and high levels of other B vitamins. Some examples of lean pork products are pork loin or veal. Lean beef, which is any beef that contains less than 10 grams of fat, are great sources of B vitamins, iron, and magnesium. Some examples of lean meats are ground round, ground sirloin, or 90% lean ground beef. You can healthily cook lean pork or beef by broiling, grilling, or roasting it. Lean meats pair best with fresh vegetables, brown rice, or whole grain pasta for a super energizing meal.

Skinless Chicken

Skinless chicken contains loads of protein, magnesium, and B vitamins, making it an excellent food source for energy. Best of all, skinless chicken is very versatile. You can cut it into strips for a salad, you can make it into a sandwich topped with delicious, energy-boosting vegetables, or you can have it as your main dish with a side of fresh vegetables or brown rice.

Clams

Clams are a type of shellfish that has high levels of iron. Clams also generally contain at least 30% of the recommended serving of iron for our bodies and contain high levels of Vitamin B12. They are a good food option for those who really like eating seafood. Many grocery stores carry frozen or canned clams. The most popular way to cook clams is to steam them, which only takes a few minutes.

Oysters

Oysters are another type of shellfish, similar to clams, which contain around 30% of the recommended serving of iron for our bodies. You can steam oysters the same way you steam clams or you can cook them on a grill.

Salmon

Salmon is the best type of seafood to eat for natural energy. It is low in fat, contains omega-3 fatty acids (which contain energy-boosting nutrients that the body cannot naturally produce), and high levels of protein. Salmon makes a great energy-boosting, main course dinner, especially when paired with whole grain pasta, brown rice, or a delicious vegetable like asparagus or spinach. You can bake, broil, or grill salmon for a healthy source of natural energy.

Beans

Not only are beans a great side dish or side ingredient but they are also great for providing our body with energy. Beans are a powerful food as they come packed with low-fat proteins, iron, magnesium, and Vitamin B12. There are also many kinds of beans to choose from. You can eat baked beans with hot dogs, turn garbanzo beans into a healthy hummus dip, or add pinto beans to a pasta dish.

Whole Grain Pasta

Whole grain pasta is a great, healthy, and energetic alternative to regular pasta. It is packed with complex carbohydrates and fiber so your stomach will digest it slowly. It also contains iron, protein, and magnesium, all of which will provide your body with natural energy. You can eat pasta with vegetables, sauce, meat, or as a side dish.

Asparagus

Green vegetables are a great source of energy. Not only will asparagus provide your body with all the B vitamins it needs, it allows you to stay energetic throughout the afternoon and evening. As a bonus, it also protects against cancer, which makes it a great food option. A delicious and super easy way to make asparagus is to lightly cover it in olive oil and bake it at 450 degrees for fifteen minutes on a metal pan.

Sauerkraut

Sauerkraut is a great energy food because it helps your digestive system work better and faster. You will find yourself with more energy after eating sauerkraut because your body won't spend as much energy digesting it. You can eat sauerkraut by itself but many people like to use it for toppings on hot dogs, bratwurst, and kielbasa.

Fresh Spinach

Dark greens, such as spinach, are great sources of energy. Spinach provides us with up to 200% of Vitamins A and C. It also has iron, fiber, and protein, all of which are essential for healthy blood sugar levels and a healthy digestive system. You can eat fresh spinach in a salad, a wrap, as a side dish, or as a sandwich topper. Be sure to use fresh spinach and not canned spinach, as canned spinach can contain high levels of sodium.

Snacks

Yogurt

Yogurt is a great option for a snack or even for a quick breakfast. While classic yogurt has enough protein to keep your body energized, Greek yogurt is an even better option for an energizing snack. Not only does Greek yogurt contain higher levels of protein, it has less sugar (which prevents a sugar crash) and contains high levels of probiotics, which help improve your digestive system. You can buy classic yogurt and Greek yogurt in little "to-go" cups, which makes it a great on-the-go snack. It usually comes in plain or mixed with fruit. You can even buy the plain kind and add your own fruit to create a customized snack that will fill you with natural energy.

Nuts

Nuts are an easy snack and a great source of energy-boosting nutrients. Most nuts contain high levels of protein and fiber, which can stabilize your blood sugar and help your digestion. Cashews, almonds, and hazelnuts contain magnesium and are great for snacks or as part of a meal. Almonds in particular are known for giving great energy when eaten. The best thing about nuts is that you can eat them in trail mix, by themselves, or in a mixed bag. They are portable, small, and very energizing. You can also get your source of nuts by eating peanut butter. For an amazing, energy-boosting snack, spread some peanut butter and honey on a piece of whole grain bread.

Honey

Honey is a natural sweetener (much better than sugar!) and is great for building strong muscles, which leave some room in our bodies for extra energy because we don't have to exert ourselves as much. Best of all, you can use honey on almost anything. You can add it to your tea instead of using sugar or other unhealthy sugar substitutes. You can put it on plain yogurt if you really enjoy its sweet taste. You can drizzle it on almost anything for a sure-fire dose of natural energy.

Peanut Butter

Many people do not view peanut butter as a "healthy" or "energetic food source" because of its high calorie count. However, peanut butter is actually a very healthy food and an excellent way to give your body an energy-boost. Since it contains nuts, it has a high content of fiber and protein. Peanut butter also contains high levels of magnesium. The great thing about peanut butter is that many people like it and can use it in many ways. You can spread some peanut butter on a piece of whole wheat bread or on a whole wheat bagel for a healthy peanut butter and jelly sandwich and you can even add in banana slices for some extra fiber content. Drink skim milk with your sandwich to get an extra serving of protein. The store bought peanut butters tend to add a good amount of extra sugar, so if you really want to be healthy try and get the 100% natural peanut butter.

Apples

Not only are apples a great energy-boosting food, but they are small, portable, and make a great snack. They contain high levels of fiber so your body can easily digest them. There are many kinds of apples to snack on: gala, fuji, granny smith, red delicious, and golden delicious, just to name a few. You can eat apples whole or you can slice them up for a fun and easy snack. Add some peanut butter to your apple for a delicious treat.

Bananas

Bananas are a great energy-boosting food because they contain good sugars and high levels of fiber, which helps your body digest them more slowly. Bananas are a great "on the go" snack because you can carry them almost anywhere, since they are protected by their skin. You can peel the skin and eat a whole banana or slice one up for your peanut butter sandwich, cereal, or oatmeal.

Blueberries

Blueberries are small, portable, and a great food source for energy. They contain Vitamins C, E, and A, as well as niacin, which helps your body convert the vitamins into energy. Blueberries are also a great source of iron, potassium, manganese, and fiber, almost every nutrient that you need for an energetic day. Blueberries are perfect toppers for oatmeal and yogurt, great in smoothies or in jelly, or even by themselves.

Strawberries

Strawberries are like blueberries in the sense that they are small, portable, and a great food source for energy. Strawberries are unique from other fruits because they contain the highest levels of Vitamin C. They are also full of fiber, B vitamins, magnesium, and omega fatty acids. You can eat them by themselves or add them to your yogurt, oatmeal, or cereal. They also make great dessert options if you dip them in melted dark chocolate.

Dark Chocolate

Dark chocolate is a healthy choice because it contains antioxidants that help improve the functions of our heart. When our hearts are healthy and strong, they are able to pump more oxygen throughout our bodies, thus giving us more energy. It also slowly makes its way into our bloodstreams, which is good for digestion. Dark chocolate makes for a great mid-day snack or a great after-dinner dessert. Many people like to eat dark chocolate with a glass of wine. Red wine, in particular, is also great for heart health, so you can combine it with dark chocolate for extra energy. Just remember to eat dark chocolate sparingly—too much chocolate is never good for our bodies.

Popcorn

Are you the kind of person who can't watch a movie without a bowl of popcorn? If you are, good news: popcorn contains whole grains, which makes it a healthy, energizing snack. It also contains high amounts of fiber and is fun and easy to make. The best way to make popcorn is to air pop it or microwave it, if you cannot air pop it. If you're eating it at the movie theater, eat a small portion and try not to add extra butter or salt, which is generally unhealthy.

In general, try to avoid food and drinks such as energy drinks, sodas, doughnuts, glazed rolls, fast food, and alcohol. All of these are generally unhealthy and contain high levels of refined sugar, caffeine, and/or fat. Many of them can lead to more health problems in the future and can be detrimental to your sleeping patterns, especially if you're not exercising.

Three Ultimate Recipes For Energy

You can eat energy-boosting foods by themselves or combine them together to make an ultimate energy-boosting meal. This section includes three super-energizing recipes that you can make at home. They utilize many of the energy super foods from above.

Egg and Salmon Breakfast Sandwich

For a breakfast that will keep you moving throughout the day, try out this egg and salmon breakfast sandwich. What you will need is:
- Extra-virgin olive oil
- One red onion, finely chopped
- 2 large egg whites
- Salt
- Capers, rinsed and chopped (optional)
- Smoked salmon
- Sliced tomato
- 1 toasted whole wheat english muffin

Over medium heat, add ½ a teaspoon of olive oil in a pan. Add the chopped onion and stir it for a minute until it gets soft. Next, add the egg whites, salt, and optional capers and stir for 30 seconds. Toast the English muffin and add 1 ounce of smoked salmon, the egg white mixture, and a slice of tomato. For a complete breakfast and added energy, add a piece of fruit and a cup of 100% juice.

Peanut Bars

For a great, "grab and go" mid-day snack that doesn't require any cooking, try these ultimate energy peanut bars. You will need:

- Dry roasted, salted peanuts
- Roasted sunflower seeds
- Raisins
- Rolled oats
- Toasted rice cereal
- Toasted wheat germ
- All natural peanut butter (crunchy or smooth)
- Packed brown sugar
- Honey
- Vanilla extract

Apply cooking spray to a 9x13 pan. Add ½ cup peanut butter, brown sugar, and honey to a bowl that you can put in the microwave. Microwave it for 1 to 2 minutes. Add one teaspoon of vanilla extract and blend the mixture together by stirring it. Add ½ cup of peanuts and sunflower seeds, 2 cups of raisins, oats, and rice cereal and ¼ cup of wheat germ. Blend the ingredients together until the peanut butter mixture completely coats the dry mixture. Put the final mixture in the pan and let it sit. After an hour, it should be hard enough to cut into pieces.

Beef, Broccoli, Yam Stir Fry

This healthy, energy-boosting stir-fry makes a great lunch or dinner option. It brings together healthy greens, energy-boosting sweet potatoes, and all of the essential amino acids our bodies can get from lean beef. You will need:

- Water
- Packed brown sugar
- Oyster sauce
- Crushed red pepper
- Flank steak
- Corn starch
- Broccoli florets
- Red-skinned sweet potatoes
- Fresh ginger, peeled

In a bowl, combine ¼ cup of water, 3 tablespoons of sugar, 3 tablespoons of oyster sauce, and ¼ teaspoon of crushed red pepper. Stir together until the sugar dissolves and put aside. Next, cut the flank steak into 1/4-inch slices and coat with the corn starch. Over high heat, add 1 ½ tablespoons of oil to a pan and stir-fry the steak for 3 minutes. Take the steak out, reheat the leftover oil, and simmer 4 cups of broccoli florets, 8 ounces of sweet potatoes, and 2 teaspoons of fresh ginger over medium-high heat. After the vegetables cook, add the steak and sauce and toss it.

Drinks

Water

When eating a healthy meal or snack, you will probably want to know what to drink with it. Keeping your body hydrated is a great way to stay energized. The healthiest way to keep your body energized is to drink water. Water is fresh and pure, unlike sodas or energy drinks, which contain high levels of sugar. If you want to give your glass of water a little flavor, you can put a slice of lemon, orange, or lime in it. My favorite way of getting water is with the ZeroWater filtration system. You can also but the filters in bulk to save some money. ZeroWater Filters

Smoothies

Smoothies are another great drink option for good health because they contain energy-rich ingredients and they are thicker than a glass of water or juice, which will make you feel fuller. Smoothies are easy and fun to make, as long as you have a blender. The NutriBullet blender makes great smoothies.

Ultimate Berry Smoothie

For this smoothie, you will need:

- Fresh berries (blueberries and strawberries are the best kind for energy)
- Plain, low-fat yogurt
- Orange juice
- Non-fat dry milk
- Toasted wheat germ
- Honey
- Vanilla extract

Add 1 ¼ cup of the berries, ¾ cup of the yogurt, ½ cup of the orange juice, 2 tablespoons of the dry milk, 1 tablespoon of the wheat germ, 1 tablespoon of honey, and ½ a teaspoon of the vanilla extract to a blender and blend.

Banana Berry Smoothie

This very simple smoothie recipe combines lots of energizing fruit together for a feeling of mental and physical alertness. You will need:

- 1 banana
- Frozen or fresh strawberries

- Frozen or fresh blueberries
- Frozen or fresh blackberries
- Frozen or fresh raspberries
- Orange juice

Break up the banana into pieces into the blender. Then, add one cup of orange juice, 2/3 cup of a mixture of the frozen berries, and then blend until it becomes a smoothie.

Green Peanut Butter Smoothie

This smoothie includes spinach, a very energizing, dark-green vegetable. However, don't let the thought of spinach in your smoothie scare you away from this energizing smoothie. You will need:

- Milk
- Greek Yogurt
- 1 banana
- All natural peanut butter
- Fresh spinach

Add 2/3 cup milk, ½ cup of greek yogurt, the banana, 1 tablespoon of all natural peanut butter, and 2 cups of fresh spinach to your blender and blend.

Chapter 4: All Natural Vitamins and Supplements for Energy

If you have ever walked through your local pharmacy, you have probably noticed that they have a large section of vitamins and supplements specifically for boosting your levels of energy. If you decide to boost your energy using all natural vitamins and supplements, it is good to know a bit on how they work before you take them. For example, some of them may work well for some people and not for others. If you're an athlete looking to boost your athletic performance, you may benefit from one type of supplement more than a person who is looking to boost their overall daytime energy. Some experts argue that as long as you maintain a healthy diet, you will not need to use energy-boosting vitamins or supplements. However, those who have vitamin deficiencies, especially with B vitamins, can definitely benefit from these substances. I have personally been taken vitamins and supplements over the last twenty five years with great success.

The best time of day to take energy-boosting vitamins and supplements is in the morning, usually right after you eat breakfast. Taking these substances in the morning helps give your body an additional amount of energy and it also helps your body digest your breakfast better, which leaves you with some extra, unused energy for the rest of the day. Since some energy-boosting vitamins and supplements act as stimulants, it is best not to take them at night or before you go to bed, as it could lead to insomnia and have some negative effects. I recommend that you take them with a meal because the nutrients in them will digest better with the nutrients found in a healthy meal, and they will not upset your stomach if taken with food.

You can take some vitamins and supplements together if the nutrients in them work together chemically. Always consult with your doctor before taking a vitamin or supplement for energy—if you find yourself lacking energy all the time, you may have an illness that a health professional needs to address. However, if you are in pretty good health, a vitamin or supplement for energy may work just fine.

This chapter will outline the top 15 best all natural vitamins and supplements. Each one is unique in its characteristics and may work differently for different people.

Licorice Root

Licorice root is my favorite natural, energizing supplement and has worked the best for helping me feel more energized throughout the day. Studies have consistently shown that licorice root helps boost our energy levels by helping our bodies regulate stress-inducing hormones. One licorice root supplement that has worked best for me is **Nature's Way Licorice Root**. I like this product because it sells for a reasonable price and works great. You can swallow the capsules by mouth or you can break them open and add the powder to a cup of tea or water.

Oat Straw Extract

Oat straw extract is a natural substance that helps your heart pump more blood to your brain, which will give you more energy throughout the day. A really good oat straw extract is: **Iowa Select Oatstraw Extract**. This liquid is made from fresh, organic herbs and comes right from Iowa. It also comes in liquid form, which is appealing to those who do not like to swallow pills. You can put it in your juice or tea and drink it right down. If you often feel tired in the morning, this product may work well for you. I have noticed a considerable difference in waking up in the morning with more energy once I started taking this product.

Rhodiola

Rhodiola is a great natural supplement to take if you often find yourself feeling sluggish in the afternoon. This substance helps duplicate the molecules in the body that give us energy. I highly recommend the **NOW Foods Rhodiola Rosea** supplement. Unlike many herbal supplements, this brand does not have a smell or a taste, which makes it easy to take. It is also relatively cheap and you get a lot of pills for a reasonable price.

Multivitamins

Multivitamins are a great source of energy because, like their name says, you can get multiple nutrients from one pill. Most multivitamins contain all the essential B vitamins and amino acids that our bodies need for balanced health and energy. One important thing to note is that most multivitamins labeled specifically for energy often contain caffeine, so if you're looking to stay away from that stimulant, be sure to read the labels carefully. The best thing about multivitamins is that there are special types for males and females.

For men, a great multivitamin brand is **Optimum Nutrition Opti-Men Multivitamins**. This brand contains over 350 milligrams of B vitamins, amino acids, and enzymes that help your digestive system. These pills are slightly larger than average, so taking them with a glass of water may help you swallow them easier.

For women, a great multivitamin brand is **Optimum Nutrition Opti-Women Multivitamins**. This multivitamin is the same brand as the one for men, except some of the ingredients are customized for a female body. This vitamin gives women a full dose of iron, which is an essential nutrient for natural energy. Many women have reported that they feel as energetic when taking this vitamin as when they drink a cup of coffee.

Coenzyme Q10

Coenzyme Q10 is a substance that your body makes naturally as well as a substance that can come from an outside source. Coenzyme Q10 helps with an energy boost by enhancing the way that energy-producing molecules recharge in our bodies. Although our bodies produce this substance on its own, some people may have deficiencies, such as those with AIDS, heart failure, or high blood pressure. One great coenzyme Q10 supplement is **Nature's Bounty Co Q10**. This product helps support heart health while also giving an extra spurt of energy.

Ginseng

Ginseng is a natural, plant-based herb that grows in Asia and North America. Ginseng is best known for boosting the immune system and lowering sugar levels in the blood. Recently, scientists have conducted studies that showed how ginseng boosted the energy of cancer patients who received chemotherapy as well as those without cancer. One excellent brand of a natural ginseng supplement is **Irwin Naturals Ginza Plus Endurance**. The key ingredients are omega-3 fatty acids, rhodiola, and ginseng.

Vitamin B Supplement

As you already know from the chapter on energy super-foods, B vitamins are important for boosting our levels of energy. Although we can get a percentage of B vitamins through the foods we eat, we can also get them in the form of a supplement. This is especially good for people who may have any B vitamin deficiencies. One of the best B vitamin supplement products is **Nature Made Super B Complex Tablets**. For less than $10, you get 360 tablets that provide your body with all eight B vitamins that your body needs for a burst of energy. You can take these vitamins with a multivitamin for an extra boost of energy. Vitamin B-12 is also famous for increasing energy levels and a highly recommended supplement. A good B-12 supplement is: **Jarrows B-12**. It is chewable and tastes great.

Amino Acids

Amino acids help your body stay energized throughout the day—without them, our energy will drain right out from under us. We can provide our bodies with amino acids by eating plenty of protein-rich foods or we can get them in the form of a natural supplement. My favorite amino acid supplement is **Country Life Max Amino with B-6**. Four of these capsules will provide your body with all of the essential amino acids that it needs to thrive. To successfully use this product, take 2 to 4 capsules per day in between meals. To get a long energy boost that will last you throughout the day, take 2 pills after breakfast and 2 before dinner.

Another really good amino acid supplement is **Optimum Nutrition Essential Amino**. These tablets are chewable and come in different flavors, which are good for those who dislike the taste of regular pills. This supplement is especially good for a pre-workout energy boost and is my personal favorite.

Bee Pollen

Bees make bee pollen naturally and it is a great source of all the nutrients that the human body needs. 40% of bee pollen is protein while the rest of it is amino acids and B vitamins. Bee pollen is great for building up stamina and staying energetic. One good bee pollen supplement is **Nature Cure Bee Caps**. This product brings together the best bee pollen from all around the world as well as including royal jelly, which can help your body recharge. You can take the capsules by chewing them or swallowing them with water. Highly recommended.

Spirulina

Spirulina is a plant that thrives in water and has a texture that is similar to seaweed. Though it is similar to algae, it is actually very healthy for the body and good for energy because spirulina contains high levels of protein. You can take spirulina through a supplement. A great spirulina supplement is **Emerald Energy Defense**. The formula in this supplement promotes good health in general to keep your physical and mental energy levels consistently high. You can stir this substance into a glass of cold milk or juice every morning with breakfast.

Gotu Kola

Gotu Kola is a natural substance that countries like China and India have used to improve mental focus. It comes from a plant and does not contain any caffeine. If you often suffer from stress and anxiety, gotu kola may be able to help you relax and clear the fog from your head. A great way to take gotu kola is to take **Nature's Way Gotu Kola**. This product comes with 100 capsules for less than $10. The best way to take this supplement is to take one capsule with a heavy meal. It can be with breakfast or lunch, depending on when you feel the most sluggish.

Iron

As you know from the section on foods, iron is one nutrient that helps our bodies produce energy. If you do not wish to get iron by eating iron-rich foods, you can take it in the form of a supplement. One of the top supplements for iron is **Nature Made Iron**. These capsules are free of any artificial substances or preservatives and are small, making them easy to swallow. This brand also comes at a great price.

Omega-3 Fatty Acids

As you have also learned from the foods chapter, omega 3-fatty acids are another natural substance that helps your body stay energized. However, the best way to get this substance is to eat seafood and many people are allergic or just don't have the taste for fish. The good news is that you can still provide your body with omega-3 fatty acids without actually eating seafood. One of the top supplements for omega-3 fatty acids is **Kirkland Signature Natural Fish Oil**. This supplement combines nutrients found in anchovies, herring, and salmon that are straight from the ocean. Best of all, this brand comes with 400 gel capsules for a low price of only $13, so it will last you a long time. Like many other pills, you can take these with a glass of water or juice.

Chapter 5: Living One Super-Energizing Life

By combining some or all the techniques that this book covers, you can easily help your body gain more levels of energy in no time. The first thing you should do to live an energizing life is to start making some simple changes in your life.

One way you can do this is to plan out each week. Look at your schedule and decide when and where you can exercise. Try to schedule your exercise into time frames when you can be outside in the sunlight. Exercise is a great way to naturally stimulate energy and it also leads to a good night's sleep, which will lead to even more energy. For example, you can take brisk walks in the morning, practice deep breathing in the afternoon, and do some yoga poses before bed. If your life is so busy that you truly do not have much time at all for exercise, start making wiser choices, such as taking the stairs instead of the elevator or parking further away from your destination and walking.

Next, you should reevaluate your sleeping situation. Figure out if you have the right kind of bed bedding that does not disturb your sleep. You may need to make changes in your sleeping habits, such as turning out the lights or turning off electronics. You may even want to move your bed into an area that is extra dark and quiet.

Try to expand your mind and give meditation a go. Meditation works differently for everyone, so as long as you can relax, it will most likely work for you. It's also a great way to balance and reset your mental clarity. If meditation is quite your thing, guided hypnosis sessions can be excellent. **Hypnosis Downloads** has some great programs that you can download right on your computer and listen to on your favorite audio device. **Natural Energy Booster** is a great choice for getting more energy in your life!

In terms of eating, commit yourself to buying some of the healthy options that are described in Chapter 3. Eliminate any junk food from your diet and don't even keep it in the house—it may be too tempting. Drink plenty of water and carry bottled water with you throughout the day. Try to come up with healthy combinations so you do not get tired of eating the same kinds of foods. Also, make it a point to begin reading the labels and nutrition information on everything you buy to make sure that it is free of refined sugar, caffeine, and anything else that may drain your energy. I know caffeine withdrawal can be pretty terrible, but after 4-7 days with no caffeine you should really notice that you have more energy and feel much better. I have tried many times to incorporate caffeine into a healthy lifestyle, and it just never seems to work out over the long term. I have been much more productive with great energy levels after giving up on caffeine and taking the supplements mentioned earlier.

Finally, you should talk to your doctor about your health. Find out if you have any vitamin deficiencies that may require you to start taking a natural supplement. If you decide to start taking any vitamins or supplements even if you do not have any deficiencies, you should still consult with your doctor to make sure that the decision is right for your body.

As long as you commit yourself to sticking to a new, energizing lifestyle, you will begin to see changes in your body and your life very quickly. If you have trouble committing yourself to something, please check out my book **Influence, Willpower, and Discipline**.

Here are some other tips that you can use to become more energetic:

- Surround yourself with positive people. Good energy is contagious just as much as bad energy is. By surrounding yourself with positive, uplifting people, you will feel it in yourself.
- Drink water consistently.
- When you're feeling down, depressed, and unmotivated, listen to some uplifting music for a quick, mental energy fix, and don't forget the deep breathing exercises.

I used to live a very draining lifestyle. I didn't think that I had much time to exercise and eat right. I also had no idea that my sleeping situation was leading to my loss of energy. I used to get up in the morning, go to work, and then come home exhausted. I barely had any time to spend with my family and friends. Then, I started to make some changes in the way I took care of my body. After making exercise a priority, switching out processed foods for more natural and healthy foods, eliminating caffeine, and taking energy boosting vitamins and supplements, I started to see a major change. I found myself more awake and motivated. I very rarely got exhausted and burnt out like I used to and life was that much more exciting and enjoyable. By following the advice in this book I hope you too will begin to lead a more energetic and happier life! Once you have boosted your energy levels, a great companion to go along with your increased energy is my bestselling book: **Ultimate Productivity**.

Conclusion

I hope that this book was able to help you to recognize any changes that you need to make in your daily routine in order to live a more energetic, productive, and fulfilling life.

The next step is to determine which of these steps you need to take. Start by thinking of anything that may be physically or mentally draining your energy and then use this book as a reference guide on how to overcome it. You may be surprised to see how easy it is to take steps toward improving your energy. If you have the money, the vitamins and supplements work incredibly well and don't leave you with that jittery feeling other so called energy supplements can give.

Finally, if you discovered at least one thing that has helped you or that you think would be beneficial to someone else, be sure to take a few seconds to easily post a quick positive review. As an author, your positive feedback is desperately needed. Your highly valuable five star reviews are like a river of golden joy flowing through a sunny forest of mighty trees and beautiful flowers! *To do your good deed in making the world a better place by helping others with your valuable insight, just leave a nice review.*

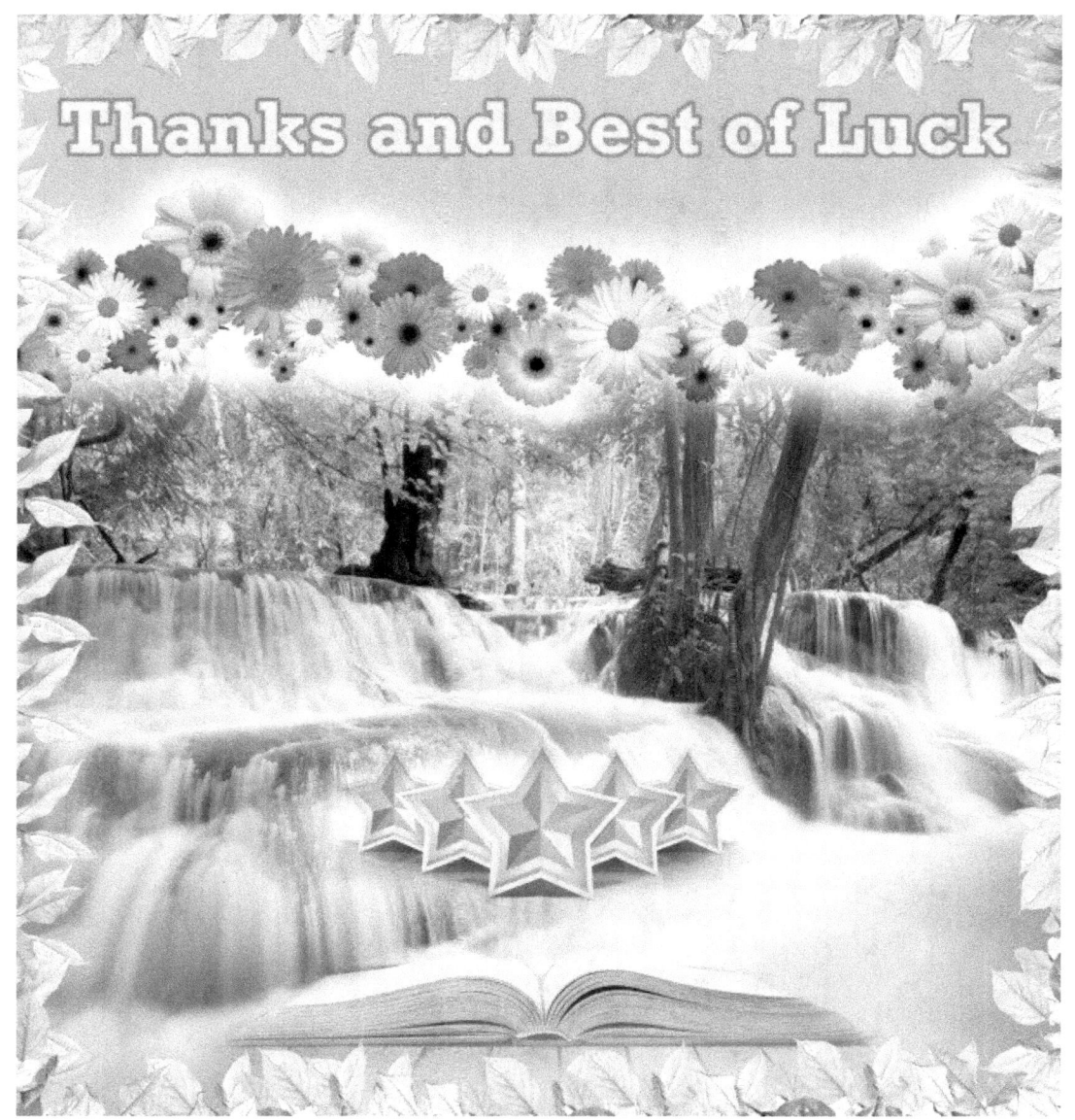

My Other Books and Audio Books
www.AcesEbooks.com

Health Books

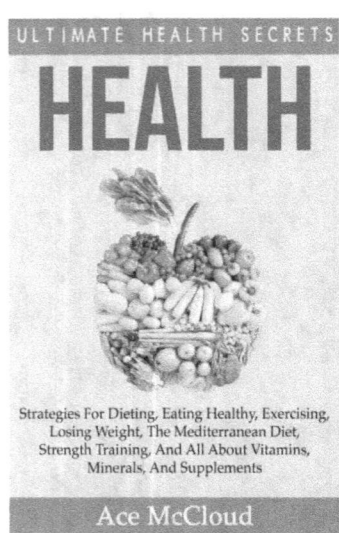
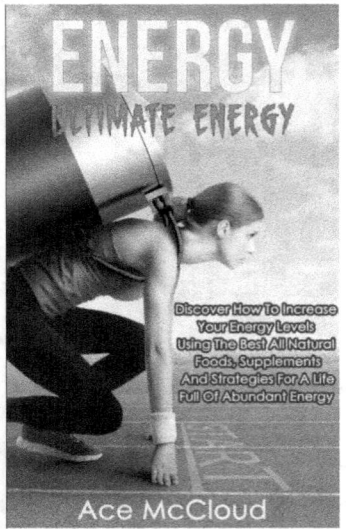
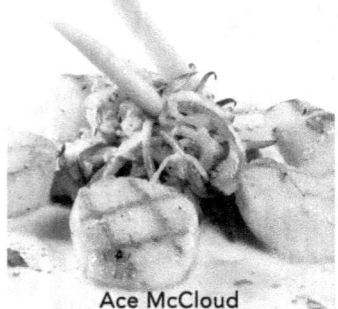
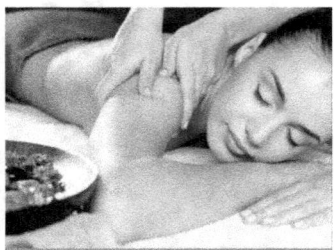
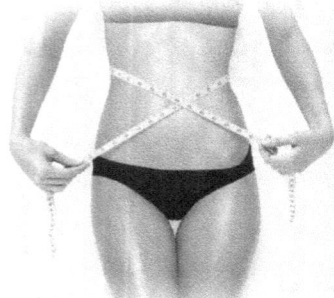
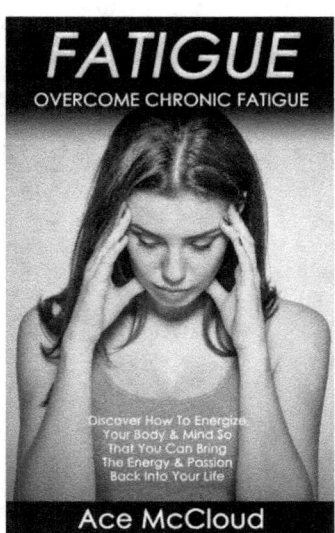

Peak Performance Books

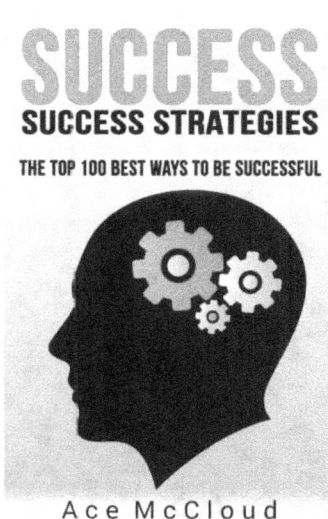
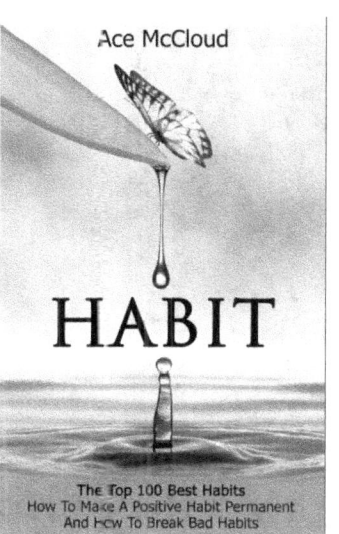
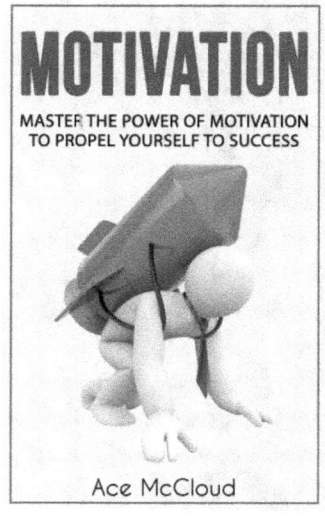
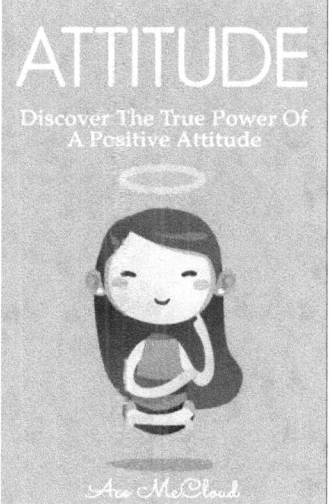

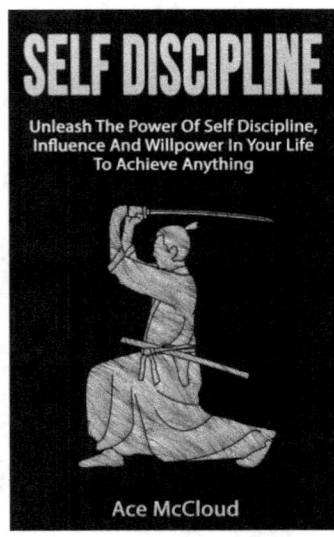 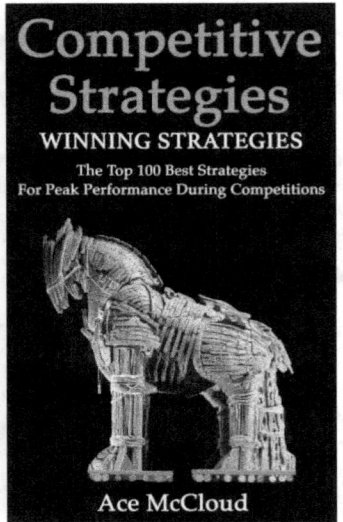

Be sure to check out my audio books as well!

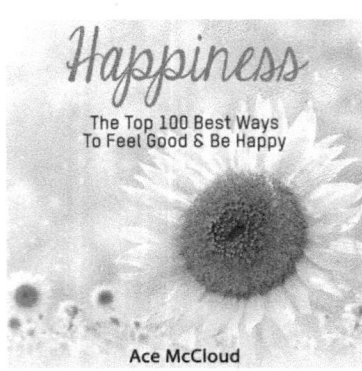 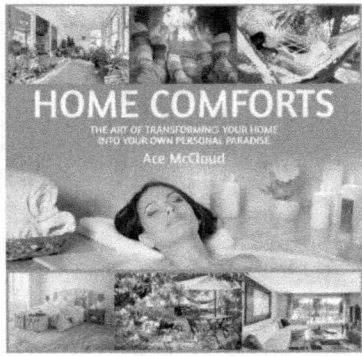 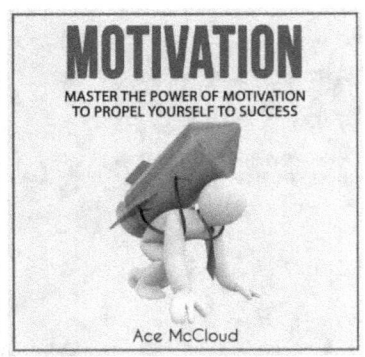

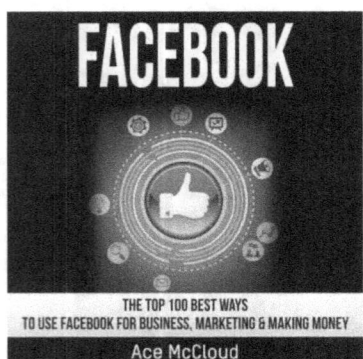 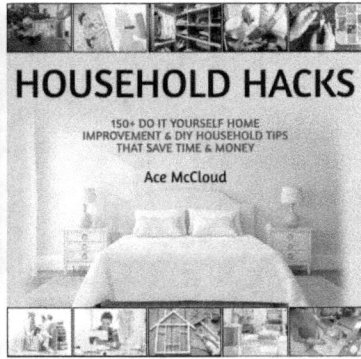 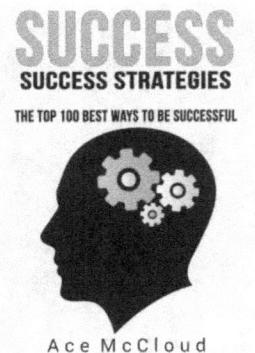

Check out my website at: **www.AcesEbooks.com** for a complete list of all of my books and high quality audio books. I enjoy bringing you the best knowledge in the world and wish you the best in using this information to make your journey through life better and more enjoyable! **Best of luck to you!**

www.ingramcontent.com/pod-product-compliance
Lightning Source LLC
Chambersburg PA
CBHW051427070526
44584CB00023B/3614